The 30-day PCOS diet plan for beginners

A 30-Day Culinary Journey to Combat PCOS and Embrace Vibrant Health with Delicious, Hormone-Balancing Recipes

Marion L. Gilley

TABLE OF CONTENT

Introduction

Polycystic Ovary Syndrome (PCOS) is a complex hormonal illness that affects many women. It is distinguished by irregular menstrual periods, elevated testosterone levels, and ovarian cysts. Along with these symptoms, PCOS frequently causes concerns with weight control, insulin resistance, and fertility. While PCOS cannot be treated, its symptoms can be effectively managed with lifestyle adjustments, such as food alterations.

Understanding PCOS and Dietary Implications: PCOS is frequently associated with insulin resistance, in which the body's cells become less responsive to insulin, resulting in high insulin levels. This can lead to weight gain, particularly in the abdomen, and raises the risk of developing type 2 diabetes. Furthermore, high levels of androgens (male hormones) in women with PCOS can cause symptoms like acne, and excess face and body.

WEEK 1: BUILDING A FOUNDATION

Polycystic Ovary Syndrome (PCOS) is a complex hormonal illness that affects many women. It is distinguished by irregular menstrual periods, elevated testosterone levels, and ovarian cysts. Along with these symptoms, PCOS frequently causes concerns with weight control, insulin resistance, and fertility. While PCOS cannot be treated, its symptoms can be effectively managed with lifestyle adjustments, such as food alterations.

Understanding PCOS and Dietary Implications: PCOS is frequently associated with insulin resistance, in which the body's cells become less responsive to insulin, resulting in high insulin levels. This can lead to weight gain, particularly in the abdomen, and raises the risk of developing type 2 diabetes. Furthermore, high levels of androgens (male hormones) in women with PCOS can cause symptoms like acne, and excess face and body.

Days 1-3: Introduction to PCOS-friendly Foods

The first three days of this 30-day PCOS diet plan are dedicated to exposing you to a variety of PCOS-friendly foods that have been specifically picked to support hormonal balance, control insulin levels, and improve overall well-being. These foods are nutrient-dense, low in processed sugars and carbohydrates, high in fiber, and contain healthy fats and proteins. By including these foods in your meals, you can create the groundwork for a healthier diet that is conducive to PCOS symptom control. The first three days of this 30-day PCOS diet plan are dedicated to exposing you to a variety of PCOS-friendly foods that have been specifically picked to support hormonal balance, control insulin levels, and improve overall well-being. These foods are nutrient-dense, low in processed sugars and carbohydrates, high in fiber, and contain healthy fats and proteins.

By including these foods in your meals, you can create the groundwork for a healthier diet that is conducive to PCOS symptom control.

Leafy Greens:

- Leafy greens are high in vitamins, minerals, and antioxidants. Examples include spinach, kale, Swiss chard, and collards.

- Add leafy greens to salads, stir-fries, smoothies, and omelets.

Cruciferous Vegetables:

- Cruciferous plants such as broccoli, cauliflower, Brussels sprouts, and cabbage contain chemicals that help the liver detoxify and regulate hormone levels.

- Cruciferous vegetables are delicious roasted, steamed, or sautéed as a side dish, or they can be added to soups, stews, or casseroles.

Lean Proteins:

- Lean proteins like chicken breast, turkey, fish, tofu, and tempeh include important amino acids that promote muscle growth and repair.

- Grill, bake, or sauté lean proteins and serve with a variety of veggies and nutritious grains.

Whole Grains:

- Whole grains such as quinoa, brown rice, oats, and barley are high in fiber, which improves digestion and increases satiety.

- Replace refined grains with whole grains in salads, grain bowls, stir-fries, or as a side dish to accompany your meals.

Healthy Fats:

- Avocados, nuts, seeds, and olive oil are rich in important fatty acids, which help with hormone production and inflammation reduction.

- To incorporate healthy fats into your diet, add avocado slices to salads, nibble on nuts and seeds, or drizzle olive oil over roasted veggies.

Low-Glycemic Index Fruits:

- Low-glycemic index fruits, such as berries, apples, pears, and citrus fruits, are less prone to produce blood sugar increases.

- Low-glycemic index fruits can be eaten as snacks, blended into smoothies, or topped with yogurt or porridge.

During the first few days, experiment with several PCOS-friendly foods and recipes to see which ones you like best. By progressively introducing these nutrient-dense foods into your diet, you can start to see positive results that benefit your overall health and well-being while effectively treating PCOS symptoms.

Day 4-7: Creating a meal plan for the week ahead

During days 4–7 of this 30-day PCOS diet plan, the emphasis switches to developing a systematic meal plan for the coming week. Meal planning is a strong tool for making informed food choices, staying organized, and maintaining dietary consistency, all of which are necessary for properly treating PCOS symptoms. By carefully planning your meals, you can ensure that you're consuming a balanced diet that supports hormonal balance, manages insulin levels, and promotes overall well-being.

Identify Your Nutritional Needs:

- Consider your unique nutritional requirements depending on age, gender, exercise level, and any dietary preferences or limits.

- Determine your calorie needs and macronutrient ratios (carbohydrates, protein, and fat) to help guide your meal planning.

Plan Balanced Meals:

- Aim to create balanced meals that include a combination of lean proteins, complex carbohydrates, healthy fats, and fiber-rich foods.

- Incorporate a variety of PCOS-friendly foods such as leafy greens, cruciferous vegetables, lean proteins, whole grains, healthy fats, and low-glycemic index fruits into your meals.

Batch Cooking and Meal Prep:

- Consider batch cooking and meal planning to save time and make meal preparation easier throughout the week.

- Choose recipes that can be readily scaled up to make larger amounts, then separate them into individual containers for quick and easy meals.

Include Snacks:

- Plan healthful snacks to keep you full between meals and prevent overeating.

- Choose nutrient-dense snacks like Greek yogurt with berries, sliced veggies with hummus, nuts, and seeds, or homemade energy balls made from oats and nut butter.

Be Flexible:

- Be flexible with your meal plan and allow room for adjustments based on your schedule, availability of ingredients, and personal preferences.

- Don't hesitate to swap out ingredients or meals if needed, as long as they still align with your PCOS-friendly dietary goals.

Stay Hydrated:

- Remember to stay hydrated throughout the day by drinking water or herbal teas, as adequate hydration is essential for overall health and well-being.

Monitor Portion Sizes:

- Pay attention to portion sizes to avoid overeating and ensure that your meals have a healthy nutritional balance.

- Use measuring cups, spoons, or a food scale to correctly portion your food, especially when experimenting with new recipes or cuisines.

By making a planned food plan for the upcoming week, you set yourself up for success in treating your PCOS symptoms through diet. This proactive strategy helps you stay organized, make smarter food choices, and keep your diet consistent, all of which contribute to better overall health and well-being.

WEEK 2: BALANCING HORMONES

The second week of this 30-day PCOS diet plan focuses on hormone balance, specifically the underlying hormonal imbalances that are typically associated with PCOS. Incorporating anti-inflammatory foods and regulating insulin levels through diet can help balance hormone production and reduce symptoms linked with PCOS.

Day 8-10: Incorporating anti-inflammatory foods

During days 8-10 of this 30-day PCOS diet plan, the emphasis turns to introducing anti-inflammatory items into your diet.

Chronic inflammation is thought to play a role in the development and progression of PCOS, causing insulin resistance, hormonal abnormalities, and other symptoms. By incorporating anti-inflammatory foods into your diet, you can help lower inflammation in the body and potentially relieve PCOS symptoms. Here's how to include anti-inflammatory substances in your diet during this time:

Introduction to Anti-inflammatory Foods:

- Begin by learning about common anti-inflammatory foods that can help lower inflammation in the body. These foods contain antioxidants, phytochemicals, and omega-3 fatty acids, which have been found to have anti-inflammatory qualities.

Include Omega-3 Fatty Acids:

- Include foods high in omega-3 fatty acids in your diet, such as fatty fish (salmon, mackerel, sardines), flaxseeds, chia seeds, and walnuts.

- Try mixing flaxseed or chia seeds into smoothies, salads, or cereal, and include fatty fish in your dinner rotation at least twice a week.

Emphasize Fruits and Vegetables:

- Include omega-3 fatty acid-rich foods in your meals, such as fatty fish (salmon, mackerel, sardines), flaxseeds, chia seeds, and walnuts.

- Try incorporating flaxseed or chia seeds into smoothies, salads, or cereal, and include fatty fish in your dinner rotation at least twice each week.

Choose Whole Grains:

- Include omega-3 fatty acid-rich foods in your meals, such as fatty fish (salmon, mackerel, sardines), flaxseeds, chia seeds, and walnuts.

- Try incorporating flaxseed or chia seeds into smoothies, salads, or cereal, and include fatty fish in your dinner rotation at least twice each week.

Use Anti-inflammatory Herbs and Spices:

- Include anti-inflammatory herbs and spices in your recipes, such as turmeric, ginger, cinnamon, and garlic.

- Use these herbs and spices to add flavor to your dishes while also increasing their anti-inflammatory benefits.

Include Healthy Fats:

- Continue to consume healthy fats like avocados, olive oil, nuts, and seeds in your meals.

- These fats aid in reducing inflammation and promote general health and well-being.

Stay Hydrated:

- Drink plenty of water throughout the day to stay hydrated and help the body's natural detoxification process.

- Consider integrating herbal teas like green tea, which are high in antioxidants and can help reduce inflammation.

Including anti-inflammatory items in your meals from days 8 to 10 of this PCOS diet plan can help reduce inflammation in the body and improve your general health and well-being. These foods include critical nutrients and antioxidants that can aid with PCOS symptoms and hormonal balance.

Days 11-14: Managing Insulin Levels through Diet

During days 11-14 of this 30-day PCOS diet plan, the emphasis is on lowering insulin levels with dietary techniques. Insulin resistance is a typical aspect of PCOS, in which the body's cells become less responsive to insulin, resulting in high insulin levels in the blood. High insulin levels can exacerbate PCOS symptoms including weight gain, irregular menstrual periods, and hormonal abnormalities. You can enhance insulin sensitivity and control your PCOS symptoms by following particular dietary guidelines. Here are some ways to include in your diet during this period:

Emphasize Low Glycemic Index (GI) Foods:

- Consume foods with a low glycemic index, which causes blood sugar levels to rise more slowly and gradually than high glycemic index foods.

- Include low-GI foods in your diet, such as non-starchy vegetables, legumes, whole grains, and fruits like berries, cherries, and apples.

Balance Carbohydrates with Protein and Healthy Fats:

- Combining carbohydrates with lean protein and healthy fats slows glucose absorption into the system and helps to reduce insulin spikes.

- For breakfast, try whole grain toast with avocado and scrambled eggs, or for lunch, try a salad with grilled chicken and quinoa.

Limit Refined Carbohydrates and Sugars:

- Reduce your consumption of refined carbohydrates and sugars, such as white bread, rice, sugary snacks, and processed foods.

- Choose whole grains such as brown rice, quinoa, and oats, and use natural sweeteners like honey or maple syrup in moderation.

Include Fiber-Rich Foods:

- Include fiber-rich foods in your meals to slow digestion and maintain stable blood sugar levels.

- Choose high-fiber foods including vegetables, fruits, legumes, and whole grains to increase insulin sensitivity.

Eat Regular, Balanced Meals:

- Maintain consistent meal times and aim for balanced meals that contain carbohydrates, protein, and healthy fats.

- Avoid missing meals, as this might result in unstable blood sugar levels and overeating later in the day.

Control Portion Sizes:

- Portion sizes should be considered to avoid overeating and to manage calorie intake, both of which can affect insulin levels.

- Avoid overeating by using smaller dishes, measuring servings, and paying attention to hunger and fullness cues.

Stay Hydrated:

- Drink enough water throughout the day to stay hydrated and promote metabolic health.

- Limit sugary beverages and instead drink water, herbal teas, or infused water to stay hydrated.

These dietary methods are intended to promote general health and well-being while effectively controlling the metabolic components of PCOS.

WEEK 3: MANAGING WEIGHT AND ENERGY

During week three of this 30-day PCOS diet plan, the emphasis changes to weight management and energy levels, which are sometimes difficult parts of living with PCOS. Weight control is critical for people with PCOS since extra weight can aggravate symptoms including insulin resistance and hormone abnormalities. Furthermore, many people with PCOS have swings in energy levels as a result of hormone imbalances and other causes. This week's focus is on developing measures that promote healthy weight management and constant energy levels. Here's how you may improve your weight and energy management throughout week three:

Portion Control and Mindful Eating:

- Portion control involves paying attention to serving amounts and avoiding overeating.

- Incorporate mindful eating techniques, such as eating deliberately, appreciating each bite, and paying attention to hunger and fullness signals.

- Try to fill half of your plate with veggies, one-quarter with lean protein, and one-quarter with whole grains or other complex carbohydrates.

Balanced Macronutrients:

- Make sure your meals are balanced with a variety of carbohydrates, proteins, and healthy fats.

- Choose complex carbs like whole grains, fruits, and vegetables, which provide long-lasting energy and fiber to keep you satisfied.

- Include lean proteins like chicken, fish, tofu, and lentils to help with muscle growth and repair.

- Healthy fats from avocados, nuts, seeds, and olive oil will help you stay full while also providing necessary fatty acids.

Regular Physical Activity:

- Incorporate regular physical activity into your daily routine to aid with weight management and energy levels.

- The American Heart Association recommends that you engage in at least 150 minutes of moderate-intensity aerobic activity or 75 minutes of vigorous-intensity activity every week.

- Choose activities that you enjoy, such as walking, cycling, swimming, or dancing, and incorporate them into your normal schedule.

Balancing Hormones through Exercise:

- Strength training and yoga are two activities that can help you balance your hormones.

- Strength training exercises can help build muscle mass, which improves insulin sensitivity and aids in weight management.

- Yoga and other mind-body practices can help alleviate stress and promote hormonal balance.

Adequate Sleep:

- Prioritize getting enough sleep every night, as insufficient sleep can affect hormone levels, leading to weight gain and weariness.

- Aim for 7-9 hours of quality sleep per night, and stick to a consistent sleep routine.

Hydration:

- Maintain hydration by drinking plenty of water throughout the day.

- Dehydration can cause exhaustion and lower energy levels, therefore drinking plenty of water is vital for overall health and well-being.

Stress Management:

- To reduce stress, try practices like mindfulness meditation, deep breathing exercises, or journaling.

- Chronic stress can lead to weight gain and hormone disruption, so it's critical to incorporate stress-relieving activities into your daily routine.

During week 3 of this PCOS diet plan, you can use measures to promote healthy weight control, maintain consistent energy levels, and improve overall well-being. These lifestyle changes, like as portion control, regular physical activity, appropriate sleep, hydration, and stress management, can help reduce PCOS symptoms while also promoting overall health and vitality.

Days 15-17: Portion Control and Mindful Eating for Weight Management

On days 15-17 of this 30-day PCOS diet plan, the emphasis is on establishing portion control and mindful eating behaviors to aid with weight management. Many people with PCOS struggle to maintain their weight because of insulin resistance and hormonal abnormalities. Portion control and mindful eating can help you regulate your food intake, enhance satiety, and support your weight management goals. Here's how to integrate these techniques into your daily routine during this time:

Understanding Portion Control

Portion control entails being careful of how much food you eat at each meal and snack. Instead of calculating calories, try visually assessing portion sizes with your hand or everyday objects as a reference. For example, a serving of protein should be the size of your palm, a serving of carbohydrates should be the size of your fist, and a meal of fats should be the size of your thumb.

Practicing Mindful Eating:

- Mindful eating entails paying close attention to your food selections, eating deliberately, and savoring each bite.

- Sit at a table with no distractions, such as phones or televisions, and concentrate on the sensory sensation of eating. Examine the colors, textures, and flavors of your meal.

- Chew your food fully and pause between bites to check your hunger and fullness indicators.

Using Smaller Plates and Bowls:

- Use smaller dishes and bowls to reduce portion amounts without feeling deprived.

- Using smaller plates might fool your brain into believing you're eating more than you are, which can help you avoid overeating.

Listening to Hunger and Fullness Cues:

- Tune in to your body's hunger and fullness cues to help guide your eating habits.

- Eat when you're hungry and stop when you're full, rather than waiting until you're stuffed.

- Pay attention to bodily hunger cues like stomach growling, as well as signs of fullness like feeling content or somewhat full.

Avoiding Distractions While Eating:

- Avoid distractions like watching TV, scrolling through your phone, or working while eating.

- Eating consciously, without interruptions, allows you to concentrate on your food and detect your body's hunger and fullness signals.

Practicing Portion Control with PCOS-Friendly Foods:

- Use portion control principles with PCOS-friendly foods like lean meats, healthy grains, fruits, and vegetables.

- Be mindful of portion sizes and try to fill your plate with a variety of these nutrient-dense meals.

Staying Hydrated:

- Drink water throughout the day to stay hydrated and support your body's natural hunger and fullness signals.

- Thirst can sometimes be confused for hunger, so staying hydrated might help you avoid unneeded snacks.

During days 15-17 of this PCOS diet plan, incorporate portion control and mindful eating habits into your routine to support your weight management objectives and improve your relationship with food.

Days 18-21: Incorporating Regular Physical Activity

Days 18 through 21 of this 30-day PCOS diet plan are dedicated to encouraging regular physical activity to enhance energy levels and aid with weight management. Physical activity aids in the management of PCOS symptoms by increasing insulin sensitivity, promoting weight loss, decreasing inflammation, and improving overall well-being. Here's how to incorporate regular physical activity into your schedule during this period:

Choose Activities You Enjoy:

- Select physical activities that you enjoy and look forward to, such as brisk walking, cycling, swimming, dancing, yoga, or weight lifting.

- Participating in pleasant activities increases the likelihood of long-term adherence to your fitness strategy.

Set Realistic Goals:

- Set attainable physical activity goals based on your current fitness level, schedule, and personal preferences.

- Begin with attainable goals, such as aiming for 30 minutes of moderate-intensity exercise most days of the week, then progressively increasing length and intensity as you build strength and endurance.

- Drink plenty of water before, during, and after your workout to stay hydrated and perform effectively.

- Feeding your body nutritious foods with a combination of carbohydrates, protein, and healthy fats will provide energy for physical exercise and aid muscle repair.

- Including regular physical exercise in your daily routine from days 18 to 21 of this PCOS diet plan can enhance your energy, help you lose weight, and improve your overall health. Remember to select things that you enjoy and establish realistic

Incorporate Cardiovascular Exercise:

- Include aerobic exercises that boost your heart rate and improve cardiovascular fitness, such as brisk walking, jogging, cycling, or swimming.

- Aim for at least 150 minutes of moderate-intensity aerobic exercise or

75 minutes of vigorous-intensity aerobic exercise every week, spread out across several days.

Incorporate Strength Training:

- Include strength training sessions to increase muscle mass, metabolism, and body composition.

- Include exercises that target specific muscle groups, such as squats, lunges, push-ups, and dumbbell rows, and aim to undertake strength training at least twice a week.

Stay Active Throughout the Day:

- Look for ways to incorporate physical exercise into your daily routine, such as taking the stairs instead of the elevator, parking farther away from your destination, or going for short walks during breaks at work.

Be Consistent:

- Prioritize consistency in your physical activity routine by scheduling regular workouts and sticking to your schedule as precisely as possible.

- Consistency is key for reaping the benefits of physical activity and reaching your fitness goals.

Listen to Your Body:

- Pay attention to how your body responds to physical exertion, and adjust your routine accordingly.

- If you experience discomfort or pain, change your activity or contact a healthcare practitioner or fitness specialist.

Stay Hydrated and Fuel Your Body:

- Drink plenty of water before, during, and after your workout to stay hydrated and perform effectively.

- Feeding your body nutritious foods with a combination of carbohydrates, protein, and healthy fats will provide energy for physical exercise and aid muscle repair.

Remember to choose things that you enjoy, set acceptable goals, be persistent, and listen.

WEEK 4: SUSTAINABLE LIFESTYLE CHANGES

The fourth week of this 30-day PCOS diet plan focuses on making long-term lifestyle adjustments that improve health and well-being. Sustainable lifestyle modifications are required for effective PCOS symptom management and long-term health maintenance. In this final week, we'll look at different techniques for adding long-term behaviors into your daily routine to help you manage PCOS. Here's how to adopt sustainable lifestyle adjustments during week four:

Managing Stress:

- To lower stress, prioritize stress management strategies including mindfulness, meditation, deep breathing exercises, and yoga.

- Schedule regular self-care activities to help you relax and unwind, such as taking a bath, going for a stroll in nature, or engaging in a pastime you enjoy.

Prioritizing Sleep:

- Aim for 7-9 hours of quality sleep per night to promote hormonal balance and general health.

- Establish a consistent sleep routine by going to bed and waking up at the same time every day, including weekends.

Regular Physical Activity:

- Incorporate regular physical activity into your daily routine, aiming for at least 150 minutes of moderate-intensity exercise per week.

- Choose activities that you enjoy, such as walking, jogging, cycling, swimming, or yoga, and include them in your normal schedule.

Mindful Eating and Portion Control:

- Practice mindful eating by paying attention to your body's hunger and fullness cues, eating deliberately, and appreciating each bite.

- To avoid overeating, use smaller dishes, measure meals, and be careful of serving sizes.

Meal Prep and Planning:

- Continue meal preparation and planning to ensure you have nutritious meals and snacks on hand throughout the week.

- Set aside time each week to plan your meals, make a shopping list, and prep ingredients ahead of time to make cooking easier.

Hydration and Water Intake:

- Stay hydrated by drinking plenty of water throughout the day, aiming for at least 8-10 glasses each day.

- Carry a reusable water bottle with you to stay hydrated on the go, and make drinking water a regular habit.

Seeking Support and Accountability:

- Surround yourself with a supportive network of friends, family, or a support group that understands your PCOS experience and can offer encouragement and accountability.

- Consider consulting with a healthcare provider, nutritionist, or health coach to help you remain on track with your objectives and get assistance and support.

By adopting these sustainable lifestyle adjustments into your daily routine during week 4 of your PCOS diet plan, you can lay the groundwork for long-term success in managing your PCOS symptoms and enhancing your overall health and well-being. Remember that consistency and commitment are essential for obtaining long-term effects, so continue to prioritize your health and well-being after 30 days.

Days 22-24: Managing Stress and Its Impact on PCOS Symptoms

Days 22-24 of this 30-day PCOS diet plan are dedicated to studying the influence of stress on PCOS symptoms and implementing stress management measures. Chronic stress can exacerbate PCOS symptoms by changing hormone balance, increasing insulin resistance, and promoting emotional eating. By using appropriate stress management practices, you can reduce the harmful effects of stress on PCOS and enhance your general well-being. Here's how to manage stress throughout this period:

Understanding the Impact of Stress on PCOS:

- Inform yourself of the relationship between stress and PCOS symptoms. Chronic stress can cause high amounts of cortisol, a stress hormone that disrupts hormone balance and worsens PCOS symptoms like irregular menstrual periods, acne, and weight gain.

Identify Sources of Stress:

- Identify stressors in your life, both internal and external (e.g., work, relationships, finances) (e.g., negative self-talk, perfectionism).

- Keep a stress journal to note your stresses and their effects on your mood, energy levels, and PCOS symptoms.

Implement Stress Management Techniques:

- Deep breathing exercises, progressive muscle relaxation, meditation, or yoga can all help you relax and reduce stress.

- Regular physical activity, such as walking, jogging, swimming, or dancing, can help reduce stress and enhance mood by producing endorphins, the body's natural stress relief hormones.

Prioritize Self-Care:

- Make self-care a priority by scheduling time for things that bring you joy and relaxation, such as reading, listening to music, spending time in nature, or pursuing hobbies.

- Establish limits and learn to say no to excessive commitments or obligations that cause stress and overload.

Seek Support:

- Reach out to friends, family, or support groups for emotional support and motivation.

- Consider obtaining professional help from a therapist or counselor who can offer helpful stress management skills.

Practice Mindfulness and Positive Thinking:

- To increase present-moment awareness and lower stress reactivity, use mindfulness approaches like meditation or mindfulness-based stress reduction (MBSR).

- Challenge negative thought patterns and create a positive mindset by practicing gratitude, affirmations, and staying present in the moment.

Maintain a Balanced Lifestyle:

- Prioritize a healthy lifestyle by getting enough sleep, eating nutritious meals, and avoiding excessive caffeine, alcohol, and processed foods, which can worsen stress and PCOS symptoms.

By using these stress management measures from days 22 to 24 of this PCOS diet plan, you can effectively reduce stress, enhance hormone balance, and alleviate PCOS symptoms.

Days 25-28: Meal Prep and Planning for Long-Term Success

As you approach the end of your 30-day PCOS diet plan, the emphasis switches to meal planning and long-term success. Building lasting habits is critical for maintaining progress beyond the first 30 days and ensuring long-term success in controlling PCOS symptoms with nutrition. Here's how to integrate meal preparation and planning into your daily routine for long-term sustainability:

Reflect on Your Progress:

- Take some time to reflect on your journey over the last 25 days, including any problems you've faced, successes you've had, and lessons you've learned.

- Determine which techniques have worked best for you and where you may need to make changes or enhancements.

Evaluate Your Goals:

- Review your initial goals and objectives for following this PCOS diet plan, and evaluate your progress toward attaining them.

- Consider any new goals you might want to set for yourself going forward, whether they're linked to nutrition, fitness, or overall well-being.

Create a Sustainable Meal Plan:

- Utilize the knowledge and experience gained over the last 25 days to develop a sustainable food plan that aligns with your long-term health and wellness objectives.

- Include a range of nutrient-dense foods, balanced meals, and portion control measures in your meal plan to help with continuing PCOS management.

Implement Batch Cooking and Meal Prep:

- Incorporate batch cooking and meal planning into your weekly routine to save time and streamline meal preparation.

- Set aside time each week to plan your meals, go grocery shopping, and prep ingredients in advance, such as washing and cutting veggies, cooking grains, and portioning out proteins.

Stock Your Pantry and Freezer:

- Stock your pantry and freezer with PCOS-friendly staples and convenient meal prep goods like canned beans, frozen vegetables, whole grains, and healthy snacks.

- Consider purchasing storage containers, meal prep containers, and kitchen gadgets that can help you prepare and organize meals more efficiently.

Focus on Variety and Flexibility:

- To avoid boredom and guarantee nutritional adequacy, mix up your meals with a variety of foods, flavors, and cuisines.

- Stay flexible with your meal plan and be willing to make changes based on your schedule, preferences, and item availability.

Plan for Success:

- Anticipate probable hurdles or barriers along your trip and devise solutions to overcome them.

- Prepare for success by establishing healthy eating habits, such as carrying nutritious snacks, planning meals ahead of time when dining out, and paying attention to portion sizes.

By implementing meal prep and planning tactics into your daily routine from days 25 to 28 of this PCOS diet plan, you can develop long-term habits that promote successful nutrition-based management of PCOS symptoms. Consistency, organization, and adaptability are essential for maintaining progress and attaining your health and wellness objectives after the first 30 days.

CONCLUSION

Congratulations on finishing the 30-day PCOS diet plan for beginners! You've spent the last month working on managing your PCOS symptoms with diet and lifestyle changes. As you reflect on your journey, remember to celebrate your accomplishments, pinpoint areas of success, and acknowledge any obstacles you may have faced. This reflection is important because it allows you to learn from your experiences and make goals for future progress.

Reflecting on Progress and Goal Setting for Continued Improvement

Throughout these 30 days, you've made proactive efforts to manage your PCOS symptoms and improve your overall health. Whether you incorporate PCOS-friendly foods into your diet, practice portion control, engage in regular physical activity, or manage stress, every effort helps you on your path to optimal health. As you reflect on your accomplishments, consider setting clear, quantifiable goals for future improvement. Break your goals down into actionable steps, develop a plan of action, and stay inspired as you work toward them. Remember that change takes time and consistency, so be patient with yourself and acknowledge each step forward on your road.

Recommendations for Ongoing Support and Information

As you continue on your path to managing PCOS, it's critical to seek continuing support and information to empower yourself. Consider researching reliable websites, publications, support groups, and healthcare specialists who specialize in PCOS management. These sites can provide you with useful information, advice, and encouragement as you face the challenges and triumphs of living with PCOS. Remember that you are not alone on this road, and seeking help can significantly improve your overall well-being.

Review Message: As you get to the end of this 30-day PCOS diet plan, reflect on your progress and the lessons you've learned. Accept the positive adjustments you've made and use them as motivation to keep moving forward on your path to managing PCOS and reaching optimal health. Remember that modest actions can lead to big results, and your dedication to self-care and healthy living is admirable. Stay motivated, focused, and certain that you have the strength and resilience to conquer any hurdles that may arise. Continue to strive for success, and don't be afraid to seek help when you need it. Best wishes for ongoing success in managing PCOS and living your best life!